Intermittent Fasting

5:2 Fast Diet For Beginners

By

Clarissa Fleming

Table of Contents

Introduction

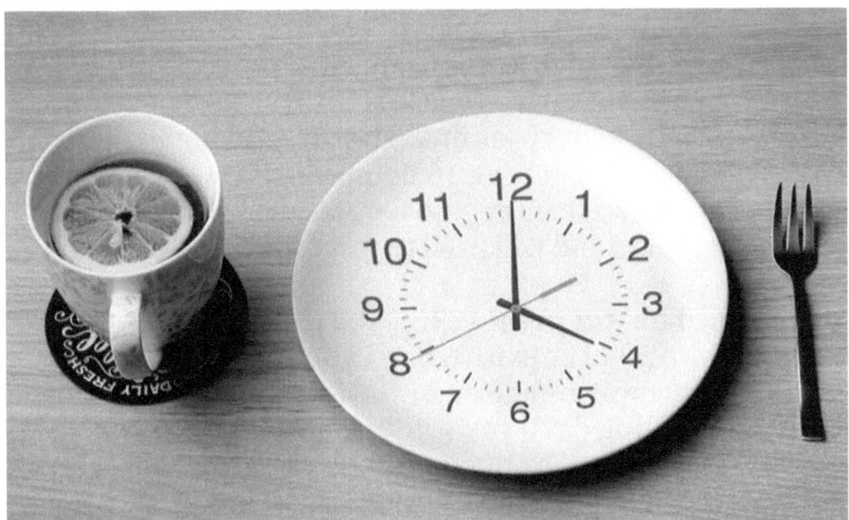

Intermittent fasting is one of the world's most popular health and fitness trends. It is not necessarily a diet, but more of an eating pattern that entails fasting for most of the day and then having your meals during a designated eating window.

Intermittent fasting does not actually change *what* you eat but rather *when* you eat. This is a crucial distinction that you need to note. People around the world are adapting to this lifestyle in order to simplify their life, improve their health, and lose weight.

Intermittent Fasting Protocols

There are a number of different ways of following this dieting lifestyle. These different ways are commonly referred to as protocols. All these protocols involve dividing the week, or day, into periods of fasting and eating. During the fasting periods, you eat absolutely nothing. You will then have all your meals during your eating window.

Common Intermittent Fasting Protocols
The following are some of the most popular intermittent fasting protocols:

1. **The 16-8 protocol:** This protocol requires you to fast for a period of 16 hours per day and then program your meals within the remaining 8-hour period. It is also known as the Leangains protocol. You can, for instance, have your first meal at 1.00 pm in the afternoon, your final meal at 9.00 pm in the evening and then fast for 16 hours. So, if you go to bed at 11.00 and wake up at 7.00 am, you will have fasted for 10 hours and will need to fast for a further 6 hours.

2. **The 5:2 protocol:** If you choose this protocol, then you will be expected to eat normally for five days of the week and fast for the remaining 2 days. During the fasting days, you will consume between 500 and 600 calories. For the rest of the week, you will eat between 2000 and 2500 calories.

3. **Eat-stop-eat protocol:** this particular intermittent fasting protocol requires you to fast for an entire 24-hour period once or maybe even twice per week. You can pick just one day of the week when you are most sedentary, then not eat anything from dinner until dinner the following evening.

There are numerous reasons why it is advisable to limit your calorie intake on a regular basis. By limiting your calories, you will most definitely lose weight. Weight is usually a factor of calorie intake. The more we eat the more likely we are to add weight. All you need to ensure is that you do not overeat during your eating windows.

Most people try intermittent fasting in order to lose weight. However, they often not only lose weight but also gain or retain muscle mass and enjoy a host of other additional health benefits.

Intermittent fasting helps you to lose weight in two ways. The first is through a reduction in calorie intake. When you consume fewer calories, you will lose weight.

You also lose weight due to hormonal changes. Since you take in fewer calories, your insulin levels are lowered significantly while the human growth hormone levels increase.

The fat-burning hormone known as noradrenaline is released into the bloodstream. Your metabolism rate will also increase. There are many positive things that work together to lose weight and also enjoy optimum health.

Chapter 1: The 5:2 Fast Diet Protocol

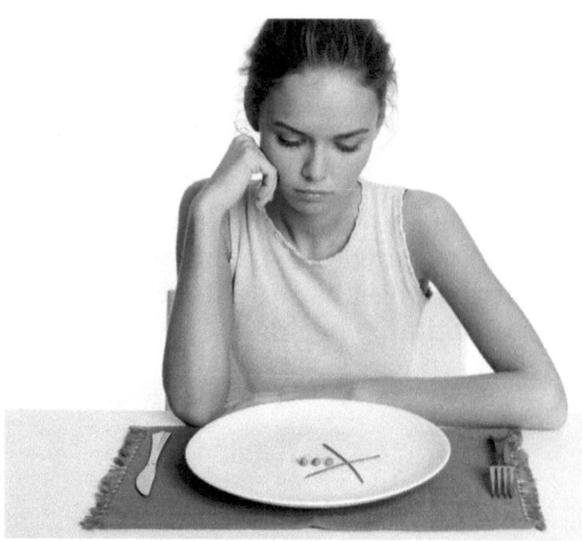

Why Do People Fail at Dieting and Intermittent Fasting?

While lots of people desire to fast because of the numerous benefits involved, many of them fail at it. People do not just fail at intermittent fasting only but also at dieting in general.

One reason that people fail is that they feel hungry and succumb to that hunger. They break the fast and are later unable to resume fasting and maintain the discipline that it requires.

A lot of dieters fail at fasting because they eat for reasons other than feeling hungry. They eat usually because of psychological and emotional reasons because they are sick or feel tired and sometimes they eat simply out of boredom.

When it comes to fasting, a lot of people are unable to maintain long hours without eating. The temptation to eat becomes too strong. Others tend to binge during their eating hours. This affects their weight loss goals. When they fail to notice any significant weight loss, they usually quit fasting and resume normal eating.

Challenging requirements

Some of the diets are rather challenging and demanding. For instance, you may be required to eat six meals per day. Other diets demand that you prepare exotic meals that may require lots of time, plenty of preparation, and rare ingredients. Other diets require that you eat plenty of fat and perhaps even raw foods. Most people are unable to keep up with these requirements.

In reality, people lead very busy and hectic lifestyles. Many do not have the time to prepare lofty diets, count calories, and so on. Some lack the budgets to spend on expensive food options. All these reasons can be summarized as follows:

- **A failure to plan:** People sometimes fail because they fail to plan. When it comes to intermittent fasting, it is crucial that you prepare your feast and fast days. You really need to plan properly, think about your meals, and find time to exercise. This is the only sure way of a successful fast diet.

- **A lack of exercise:** Regular workouts are crucial for success. Not only will regular exercises help to tone your body but will help improve your wealth, boost immunity, and definitely promote weight loss.

- **Overeating:** a lot of people who follow the intermittent fasting lifestyle often use it as an excuse to over-indulge. They often think that if they fasted for so long, they have a right to eat just about any type of food and any amount. However, this kind of thinking is completely wrong. You really should watch what you eat, including calorie intake and nutritional value of food. Eat only until you are satisfied rather than over-indulge.

- **Peer pressure:** So many times people discourage us especially when we make major decisions in life. People tend to question our choices and cast aspersions on the decisions we make. Sometimes it is advisable not to share with others some of the decisions that you make. If you

keep your plan to yourself, then you may come out
victorious more often.

- **A negative attitude:** There are times when things just
  don't work out. Sometimes it is the wrong time to try out
  new lifestyle changes or types of diet changes. For
  instance, when you are going through a life-changing
  event such as the death of a loved one, a divorce, or even
  a new job, then you may not be able to adapt to a new
  lifestyle or diet change easily.

How to Successfully Practice Intermittent Fasting

It is possible to overcome all these negative perceptions
regarding fasting and dieting. Simply ensure that you plan
ahead, drink lots of fluids, eat the right kinds of food, and get
lots of exercise. You should only share your diet and fasting
plans with important people in your life such as a friend,
spouse, or a support group that shares your interests.

One of the reasons why you can be successful with
intermittent fasting is that it is totally scientific. The idea of
restricting calorie intake and then reverting back to normal
eating triggers the body to heal, burn fat, and stimulate the
mind. That is really what intermittent fasting is all about.
Understanding and appreciating the science goes a long way
in encouraging and motivating you to keep at it no matter
how difficult it may seem at first.

1. Watch your calorie intake

Regardless of the type of diet or fast lifestyle that you choose,
calorie intake remains crucial. Calories are essential for the
body's normal functioning. However, if you take too much
then you will most likely put on weight. In order to lose
weight, you will have to start taking fewer calories.

Most other diets trigger what is known as the starvation
mode as they are usually very strict. During starvation mode,

the body slows down and you feel very hungry, confused, and even sleepy. However, with intermittent fasting, the body is made to believe that it is being overfed and hence does not enter starvation mode. However, with a calorie deficit, you will definitely lose weight.

2. Eat health foods as often as possible

Intermittent fasting is more about dividing your day or week into periods of fasting and eating. Rarely does it talk about what meals to eat and what to avoid. However, to be successful with intermittent fasting, you really should eat healthy meals as often as possible. It is okay to take the occasional cheat meal which can be something you like even though it's not as healthy such as high-calorie foods, pizza, steak, high fat, and high sugar foods. However, these should be the exception and not the rule.

Basically, processed foods are very dense when it comes to calories. This means you have to eat a lot in order to feel full. This is true, despite the fact that they contain more calories. For instance, 3 pounds of cake has a lot more calories than 3 pounds of apples.

3. Work out on a regular basis

If you are trying to lose weight, then more than eighty percent of your success will depend on the type and quantity of food that you take. However, to get the full benefits of a healthy diet, you should be physically active on a regular basis. This means you should deliberately make a choice to work out and exercise.

If you live a sedentary lifestyle, then you will not benefit much from the fast diet. The best approach to a physically active lifestyle is to identify an activity that you truly enjoy doing. For instance, if you love playing basketball, then make this your regular activity. Avoid those that you do not like because you will end up being less productive.

4. Be consistent once you get started

Another thing that you should keep in mind is consistency. With any type of lifestyle from a fast diet to healthy eating and so on, you should stick with it for some time. Basically, you will never learn whether something is bad or great for you if you do not give it some time. To find out if one of these diets and lifestyles are suitable for you, you really should give it some time. The least amount of time you should give any plan is at least 21 – 30 days.

5. Keep your lifestyle in mind

It is a fact that most people lead busy lives. Many have jobs and businesses that occupy them during the day. Some attend learning institutions like universities and colleges, while others have families to care for. It can become really challenging to pursue certain diets. For instance, you may not be able to prepare and have six meals during the day; there is basically no time for such elaborate diets and eating plans. Intermittent fasting works well for most people. It is a rewarding lifestyle that does not demand a lot from you. This means it is a suitable lifestyle even for those who are busy most of the time.

An Introduction to the 5:2 Diet

Intermittent fasting is an eating pattern that involves two distinct periods of fasting and eating. It consists of different protocols. One of the most popular protocols is the 5-2 diet. It is also known as the fast diet.

This particular protocol is the most popular of all intermittent fasting methods. It is known as the 5-2 because it allows you to eat normally for five days of the week while restricting your calorie intake on two other non-consecutive days. On these two fasting days, you will limit your calorie intake to 500 – 600 per day.

A lifestyle rather than a diet

Since you are only required to fast and eat during certain windows, this particular diet is considered more of a lifestyle than a diet. It does not dictate what foods to eat but rather when to fast and when to eat.

A lot of people find this a much easier diet or lifestyle to follow compared to numerous others. This method of eating is apparently more bearable compared to the traditional calorie-restricted diets.

On fasting days, men are limited to a total of 600 calories while women are limited to 500. You get to choose your fasting days. Try and ensure that these are not consecutive days. The most common practice is to identify days of the week when you are least active physically and with no mentally taxing activities. A lot of people prefer Mondays and Thursdays so they have carefree weekends.

You can plan to fast for 16 to 18 hours per day on your fasting days and limit your calorie intake to 500 – 600 calories. You will then have an eating window of between 6 and 8 hours. For the rest of the week, you can have regular meals and basically eat normally.

Normal eating

You need to keep in mind that while you are supposed to eat normally on the 5 non-fast days, you should not just eat anything or overindulge. If you eat unhealthy junk foods or overindulge, then you will probably not lose weight and you will not see a lot of health benefits either. Try and eat as normally as possible, choosing healthy, natural foods, and eating regular portions.

The 5:2 diet for weight loss

This fasting protocol is very effective for weight loss especially when it is done the correct way. The reason is that you will generally consume fewer calories. This is not just on your fasting day but on other days as well. Therefore, you should not try to compensate for the fasting days by overindulging on the non-fasting days.

For starters, the 5-2 diet can be just as effective as other calorie restrictive diets as long as you match the total calories. Therefore, you should not be concerned that this protocol is not as effective as other more restrictive protocols.

You can expect to lose between 3% and 8% within a period of 3 to 24 weeks. This is according to a study conducted recently by researchers. This study can be found by following this link)

https://www.sciencedirect.com/science/article/pii/S1931524 41400200X

The same study also shows that you can reduce your waist circumference by between 4% and 7% which means you are able to lose a lot of harmful belly fat through this protocol. Therefore, intermittent fasting will help you lose weight, keep you healthy and fit, and also help you maintain and possibly develop strong and lean muscle mass.

How to eat on your fasting days

Basically, there is no rule or strict requirement on what to eat or even when to eat during your fasting period. What you need to keep in mind is that you should have a fasting period and an eating window.

There are those who prefer to eat early in the morning while others prefer to wait until past midday. Different people generally have different requirements. Most people prefer having either two medium-sized meals or three small meals. These are spread throughout your limited eating window which is usually 6 to 8 hours.

Keep in mind that your calorie intake is limited to 500 or 600 calories. As such, you should split your meals accordingly. Therefore, make use of your calorie budget intelligently. As you plan your meals, you should focus on high-protein, high-fiber, nutritious meals that will keep you full even when your calorie intake is minimal.

Focus on soups and broth. These are great, especially on fasting days. Bone broth, for instance, is very nutritious and filling yet lacking in calorie content. There are plenty of other nutritious foods that you can have. They include the following:

- grilled fish
- cauliflower rice
- vegetable or tomato soup
- boiled eggs
- lean meat
- Tea
- black coffee

There is basically no right or wrong way of doing intermittent fasting. You will have to try out and experiment with lots of these meals so that you find out exactly what works for you.

On the other days when you eat normally, you should limit your calorie intake to 2000 – 2500. If you are male, then you should limit your intake to 2500 calories per day and 2000 for females.

How about when you feel unwell?

You should expect your body to react to these dietary changes. For instance, you can expect to feel weak, suffer serious hunger pangs, and basically be slower than usual and feel lethargic.

The hunger pangs will disappear pretty soon and you will be able to fast and feel normal. Also, the fasting will become a little easier after a couple of days or maybe weeks. Plenty of people attest to that.

Some people may not be used to fasting and might be doing intermittent fasting for the first time. In such a situation, you should keep a few healthy snacks like nuts for the first few days. This is in case you feel hungry but still need to maintain the fast. However, should you feel repeatedly weak, faint, or

dizzy during the fast, have something to eat and then seek
medical advice.

Chapter 2: The History of Fasting

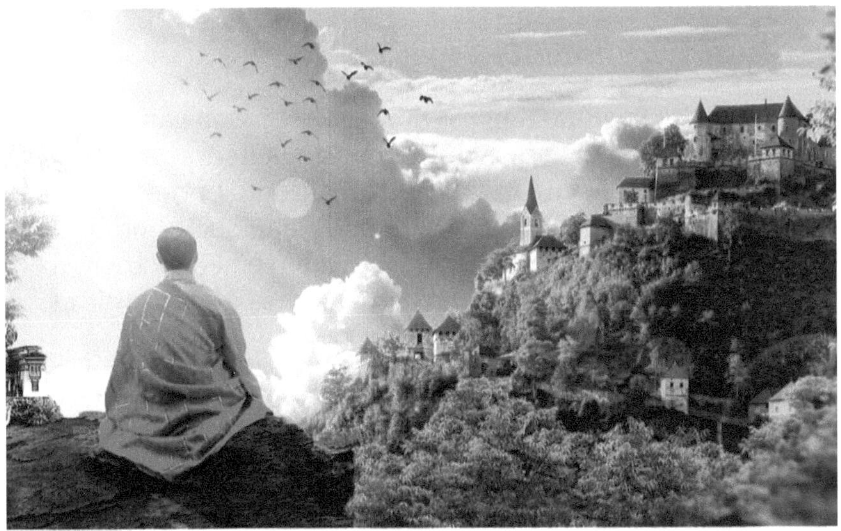

What is fasting?

Fasting refers to deliberate abstinence from drink, food, or both for a limited period of time. When you deliberately deny yourself food or drink for a couple of hours, then you will enter the fasting stage. Please note that fasting is very different from starvation.

There are plenty of different kinds of fasting practiced all over the world. One of these is absolute fasting. This is a type of fasting that requires complete abstinence from food and drink for a specific period of time such as a 24-hour period.

Time immemorial

Man has been fasting since time immemorial. Fasting has for ages been viewed by civilizations as a natural recourse when stressed or unwell. It is used a lot of the time to provide relief, rest, balance, and for energy conservation especially at critical times.

Many early philosophers, healers, and great thinkers resorted to fasting as a healing therapy. These great individuals include Plato, Socrates, Hippocrates, Galen, and Aristotle.

They have all spoken about and practiced fasting on a regular basis.

Fasting for health and religion

Man has been fasting for numerous reasons and one of these is religious purposes. Numerous ancient and modern religions advocate regular fasting. Some of these religions include Islam, Christianity, Buddhism, and Hinduism. Even Indians from across the Americas have been known to regularly fast as a part of their customs and traditions.

There are practices such as yoga that advocate the use of fasting for healing and health restoration. Ancient healing practices of Ayurveda are still practiced today as a form of therapy and for healing purposes.

Fasting in the 19th Century

Intermittent fasting was tried by health experts as far back as the early 1900s. It was used as part of a treatment regime for the treatment of obesity, diabetes, and epilepsy. This fasting lifestyle has now made a huge comeback and is very popular with different groups in our society today. Most people seeking a lifestyle that helps with weight loss management opt for intermittent fasting protocols like the 5:2 fast diet. Others with chronic conditions like diabetes and coronary heart disease choose the fast diet for health management.

Fasting is definitely not a new phenomenon to mankind. Humans have been fasting for centuries. The most common form of fasting is the typical overnight fast when we sleep. As we sleep, we do not consume any food. We only start the eating cycle upon waking up.

However, health and medical practitioners have, in the recent past, conducted clinical research studies regarding the benefits of this lifestyle. The focus has been the effect of intermittent fasting on longevity and overall health. The results have been very positive, some of which have caught the eye of healthcare experts, health enthusiasts, and many others keen on fitness and health.

There are plenty of people around the world that have quickly adapted to this exciting fasting lifestyle. They appreciate the numerous health benefits that come with it. A lot of them view this diet and lifestyle as one that people have been searching for over the decades. Most people are now taking on this lifestyle freely and there are plenty of positive reports about its benefits.

Some reasons why people choose to fast

People around the world choose to fast for a variety of reasons. According to Paracelsus, who is considered the father of modern medicine, fasting is the physician within and a great remedy for most ailments. In fact, modern medicine has recognized fasting as a great way of caring for invalids and sickly individuals. Here are some of the reasons why people choose to fast.

Health reasons – to treat ailments, diseases, and conditions

Religious reasons – some fast based on their religious beliefs

Political reasons – there are individuals who fast to try and bring attention to an issue that is important to others

Medical reasons – for purposes of medical procedures and diagnostic purposes

Fasting Versus Starvation

Food provides the body with nutrition and a source of energy. It also serves as a form of comfort. Even though food is crucial for our survival, we need to fast occasionally for health, healing, and other reasons.

It is crucial to understand the distinction between fasting and starving. Understanding the difference between the two will enable you to fast safely.

Starvation and fasting are both forms of abstinence from food. The major difference between the two is the length of time of that abstinence as well as purpose. While fasting is generally good for you, it can be harmful if prolonged.

In the absence of food in the body, chemical changes take place in our bodies that make it possible to use stored nutrients. Some of the chemicals responsible for blood regulation include glucagon, epinephrine, and insulin. They generally function together to regulate blood sugar.

When you feel hungry or enter starvation mode, your levels of epinephrine and glucagon increase while those of insulin drop significantly. The interaction between these hormones is what stabilizes blood sugar levels even as you fast. During starvation, however, all the glycogen is used up and ketones are then produced for use as an alternative source of energy. Also, protein from muscle mass is used to produce energy. When the body starts to destroy its own muscle mass, then serious consequences such as cell distortion and death are likely to occur.

Fasting basics

Fasting limits your food intake for a predefined period of time. Fasting is generally done for a number of reasons. These reasons could be for health, religion, detoxification, medical tests and so on. People usually fast for less than 24 hours when they do so for health reasons. However, this time period could be longer when done for religious reasons.

Starvation basics

Starvation is defined as a complete or severe lack of nutrition in the body necessary for maintenance and sustenance of life. Not consuming sufficient amounts vitamins, fats, proteins, carbohydrates, and minerals as well as water is considered as starvation. Starvation can have serious consequences depending on the specific nutrient deficiencies. Some of the conditions that can result due to starvation include scurvy, beriberi, and pellagra.

Differences between the two

The most basic difference between fasting and starvation is usually the severity of symptoms as well as the time between meals. Whenever you fast, you are likely to experience mild discomforts such as fatigue, headaches, dizziness, low blood pressure, and so on.

In contradiction, you are likely to experience a lot more severe side effects that include heart failure, brain dysfunction, convulsion, and possibly even death. The longer you fast, the more likely you are to enter starvation mode.

Learn to be safe as you fast

While fasting is great for you, starvation definitely is not. You need to ensure your health is never at risk. If you fast for short periods of time, then you will most likely be okay. It is advisable to speak to your healthcare provider before starting the fast diet. This is especially important if you suffer from a chronic condition such as anorexia, high blood pressure, coronary heart conditions, diabetes, cancer, and others.

As a matter of fact, most fasts lasting less than 5 days can be safely done by any individual. Those intending to fast longer than 5 days should do so under supervision by a health care expert.

Reasons for food abstinence

Fasting and starvation have different purposes. Fasting is usually done for a pre-defined period of time and for a specific purpose such as detoxification, religious reasons, and so on. On the other hand, starvation is often a result of undesirable consequences such as the inability to access nutritional food or the consequences of an eating disorder. Always take precaution whenever you embark on a calorie restriction program.

Fast Diet is a Lifestyle Rather than a Diet

Dieters who choose the fast diet make it a lifestyle rather than a diet. The reason is that if adopted, it will transform your life completely. The fast diet does not dictate what foods to eat and which ones to avoid. It merely guides your fasting hours and eating windows. One of the benefits of the fast diet is autophagy.

Autophagy

We can define autophagy as the body's most efficient recycling and detox system. It is a process that involves the repair and replacement of worn-out, old, and damaged parts. Autophagy sets in when you fast for a while. At its onset, the cells in your body create membranes that hunt down dead, diseased, and worn-out cells. These are then replaced with cell parts. Autophagy also gets rid of diseased cells as well as harmful organisms like disease-causing bacteria.

Chapter 3: How the 5:2 Fast Diet Works

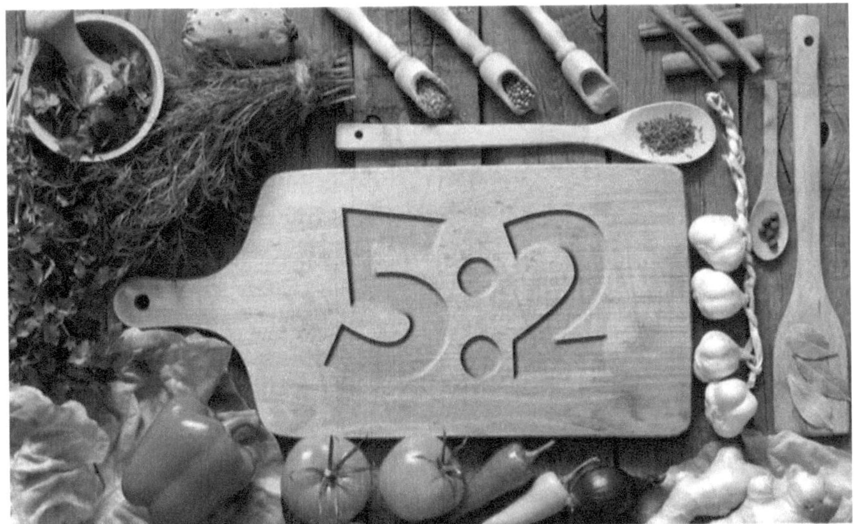

There are currently very few studies focusing on the 5-2 intermittent fasting protocol. However, there are numerous proven benefits of intermittent fasting. One of the outstanding benefits of this lifestyle is that it is much easier to follow and stick with compared to others. This is true, especially when compared to the continuous calorie diet.

Intermittent fasting has been shown to have numerous benefits pertaining to blood sugar levels. Studies show that it significantly reduces insulin levels in the body. For instance, according to this study, insulin levels can be lowered by practicing this particular diet lifestyle.

There are other studies available that also demonstrate many other benefits of the diet lifestyle. For instance, it is great for your body, your brain, and your wellbeing.

What Happens to the Body When We Fast?

When you begin fasting, you are going to feel hungry, in fact, very hungry at first. You should also expect your energy levels to drop and this might cause you to become irritable and moody. It is crucial that you prepare yourself so that you are physically and psychologically ready for the fast diet.

The body at the cellular level normally breaks down glucose in your diet to produce the energy needed to function normally. However, even as you diet, your body still needs energy. As such, the liver will begin converting amino acids and fats into glucose to produce energy. The body will then get into an energy saving mode. This results in a slowdown of body functions. Your heart rate and blood pressure will slow down and you may feel drained.

The best part is that you will only feel this way for a short period of time. After a while, your energy levels will resume as normal. As you fast, the body will go through ketosis. During ketosis, your body relies on stored fat deposits to produce energy. Once ketosis kicks in, your hunger will subside and you will then be able to proceed with your normal activities. Ketosis is great for balancing weight loss, blood sugar and so much more.

Evidence-based Benefits of the Fast Diet

1. *The fast diet alters the function of hormones, genes, and cells*

When you fast for a couple of hours, a couple of things happen within your body. These things include changes in hormone levels to ease the breakdown of stored fats and also cellular repair processes. Other changes include:

Better insulin regulation

A significant reduction in insulin levels in the blood facilitates fat burning.

The human growth hormone supply increases significantly, sometimes by up to 5 times in the body. When human growth hormone is present in larger quantities, it stimulates muscle gain and fat burning. When more fat in the body is converted into energy, there is less of it in the body.

As such, the cells and muscles become more and more responsive to insulin. The insulin becomes much better absorbed and this helps to properly regulate blood sugar. Proper regulation of blood sugar is important because it prevents conditions such as type II diabetes and better manages blood sugar for those already suffering from the condition.

Insulin resistance is a situation that is likely to happen because of excessive glucose in body tissue. This is especially true for those not designed for storage. When you fast, the stored glucose gets used up allowing your body to function normally again.

Human growth hormone

The human growth hormone, abbreviated as HGH, is responsible for causing cells in the body to divide and multiply. It helps synthesize collagen in the skeletal muscles and tendons and also boosts the immune system. HGH promotes the breakdown of lipids in the body in order to reduce body fat content while improving your physical capacity. Fasting increases HGH levels in the body and this leads to the development of strong bones, lean muscle, healthy hair growth and so much more.

Cortisol

The stress hormone cortisol is released into the bloodstream when you are stressed out. It is sometimes referred to as the flight-or-fight hormone because it triggers that exact response. Too much of this hormone in your body is not good for you. It should only be released when necessary. With your insulin properly regulated, your cortisol levels will be reduced to minimal levels.

Cells

The cells store a lot of things in them including fats and even harmful pathogens. When you fast, you trigger heightened cell activity. The body starts utilizing the stored fat and in the process also eliminated dead cells and harmful toxins and pathogens in the cells. This is basically a truly effective detoxification process that leaves you looking younger and healthier. The cells go through a repair process with new cells produced that are healthier, fat-free, and more efficient. All regular processes are then conducted very effectively and efficiently.

2. The fast diet reduces chances of type II diabetes

When you follow the fast diet, you will lower your chances of suffering from type II diabetes, which is a serious chronic condition. Plenty of people across the US and around the world suffer from type II diabetes. It occurs basically because of insulin resistance caused by excess blood sugar. When the body is unable to properly regulate insulin, a person is likely to suffer from diabetes.

The benefit of intermittent fasting is that it eliminates excess blood sugar from the cells. When the body is free from excessive blood glucose, your chances of suffering from diabetes are close to zero. Human studies have shown a reduction in blood sugar of between 3% and 6% simply through intermittent fasting. It also helps to reduce damage to the kidneys due to type II diabetes.

The fast diet reduces blood sugar levels to normal levels. Due to regular fasting, your body will process glucose much more effectively. If you are looking for a great way to regulate blood sugar, then the fast diet is one of the most effective and natural ways of achieving this objective.

3. *You will lose weight and belly fat and keep it off*

A lot of people seek long-term weight loss solutions. While there are plenty of solutions out there, none work as reliably and effectively as intermittent fasting. The fast diet is excellent for weight loss. When you fast, your body reaches your fat reserves that have accumulated over time. These fats are stored during times of plenty to be used when there is food scarcity. As such, when you begin to fast, your body embarks on a slow but deliberate weight loss process. This is immensely beneficial to your health.

If you want to lose weight in the long run, then the 5:2 fast diet is your best bet. It is a lot more effective compared to crash diets and calorie restriction diets. There are numerous studies that confirm the effectiveness of this lifestyle especially for weight loss and maintenance of optimum body weight. As you start this fast diet, you will notice considerable weight loss. With time, however, your weight will even out and you will find your optimum weight. Your optimum weight will also depend on factors such as healthy eating, regular workouts, and so on.

To add to that, the fast diet does enhance the hormones that support weight loss. These hormones support the breakdown of body fat into glucose which becomes a source of energy for the body. You will also start consuming fewer calories than before. This will come naturally to you once you get used to regular fasting. This happens even on days you are not fasting and you will not just lose weight but look and feel great as well.

One of the reasons why the fast diet is excellent for weight loss is that it works on both ends of the calorie equation. On one hand, it causes you to regularly eat less food and when you do this, you automatically lose weight. It also enhances your metabolic rate. When your metabolic rate increases, your body efficiently breaks down fat and hence less of it is stored in the body as fat.

4. Enjoy an extended lifespan

A study by the University of Chicago links the fast diet to longevity. According to scientists who conducted this research study, there is evidence showing that this dieting lifestyle delays the onset of developmental disorders that lead to death. Basically, people who fast on a regular basis get to enjoy a longer and healthier life compared to those who do not.

The aging process is hastened when your metabolism is kept busy due to regularly having three or more meals each day. Fasting provides your body a resting period. This allows cells a time to rest, detoxify, and rejuvenate. When the cells take this time out, they become a lot more efficient and this slows down the aging process.

Also, fasting puts the cells in a mild state of distress which triggers a repair-and-detoxify process. Cells that are in a state of stress will be rejuvenated and this will ensure they remain effective, efficient, and in excellent condition. These anti-aging properties of the fast diet will keep your organs functioning effectively and efficiently.

5. It boosts your immune system

One of the most important systems within your body is the immune system. This crucial system protects you against infections, diseases, and against all types of pathogens. Research scientists at the University of Southern California have clearly demonstrated how fasting regenerates the entire immune system. Fasting triggers the production of new white blood cells and these fight pathogens to keep the entire body free from diseases and infections.

The fast diet allows the body to eliminate worn out, damaged, old, and inefficient cells in your body. These are replaced by newer immune system cells. A lot of researchers think that intermittent fasting could greatly aid those prone to infection and those suffering from immunity challenges such as the elderly and sickly.

6. The fast diet is great for brain health

Scientists believe that what is great for the body is also great for your brain. This applies aptly to the fast diet because it promotes excellent brain health. When you fast for relatively short periods of time, your metabolism levels improve and this reduces blood sugar levels, oxidative stress, and inflammation.

The brain is stimulated when you fast. When this happens, it promotes the development of neurons, helps with recovery after brain injury, and enhances memory performance. The fast diet lowers the risk of degenerative brain conditions such as Alzheimer's and dementia. Intermittent fasting promotes cognitive functions and improves your quality of life well into old age.

7. It is ideal for combating oxidative stress

Free radicals constitute a major problem that we are all exposed to. These are unstable molecules that get into our bodies through varied ways such as food or drink. They are immensely dangerous to our health and can cause great harm. Free radicals are known to cause long-term damage to cells and organs in the body. They enhance the aging process and are a known precursor to dangerous conditions like cancer.

Fortunately, the fast diet provides the perfect solution because it enhances the body's protection against oxidative stress. Fasting activates stress defenses. For instance, the protein that maintains your DNA in excellent condition is activated through fasting. As you fast, the body begins to break down fats stored in your body. When this happens, waste, toxins, and dead material are also eliminated. The process also gets rid of free radicals and inflammation. When the cells are cleaned out, they get rejuvenated and become as healthy as new.

8. The fast diet benefits your heart

Heart disease is the number one killer in the USA. Millions of people across America are victims and many die of various heart diseases each year. Some of the risk factors associated with heart disease include high blood pressure, high blood sugar levels, LDL and total cholesterol, inflammatory markers, triglycerides, and others.

When you fast, you consume fewer calories than someone who is not fasting. This will result in lower levels of bad cholesterol which is absolutely good for your heart. Also, all other indicators such as inflammatory markers will improve drastically. In general, intermittent fasting has numerous heart benefits that keep your heart healthy with very low disease risks.

Benefits of Restricted Calorie Intake

Research conducted across different institutions by health experts and nutrition research scientists confirm the numerous benefits of restricted calorie intake on a regular basis. There are studies in the journal of science about research done on mice. The findings show that lifelong calorie restriction alters gut bacteria significantly. The alteration occurs in a manner that greatly supports and promotes longevity. The effect that occasional calorie restriction has on gut microbiota is longevity. It tends to lengthen the average person's lifestyle.

The Fast Diet Benefits Summary

- It limits inflammation.

- Reduces blood pressure levels.

- Improves metabolic efficiency.

- It helps to reduce oxidative stress and cellular damage.

- Prevents or slows down the progression of type II diabetes.

- Helps to reduce significant body weight in overweight and obese individuals.

- Triggers stem cells to enter into a self-renewal state.

- Improves pancreatic function.

- Modulates the levels of harmful visceral fats.

- It protects you against cardiovascular diseases.

Risks and Contraindications

Risks of fasting

One of the risks of fasting is that those who partake of this lifestyle are often dehydrated. The reason for this is that they do not obtain any fluids from food. Therefore, as you fast, you should remember to take in lots of fluids in order to keep the body hydrated.

If you were used to taking three square meals daily and snacks in between, then missing out on some of these meals and snacks will cause you increased stress. You are likely to suffer from sleep disruptions as well. Other challenges include headaches, dehydration, and possible lack of sleep.

You can also suffer from heartburns due to fasting. When there is no food in your system, your stomach acid levels will reduce. These acids usually digest food and kill off bacteria.

Sometimes though, when you smell good food, the brain may trigger the stomach to produce acid which can lead to heartburn.

A lot of nutritionists believe that the fast diet provides an excellent way to lose weight. However, there are health professionals who do not believe that this diet is beneficial in the long run. They don't think that this diet is effective for long-term weight loss. Their thinking is that fasting causes you to lose fluid quickly but not actual weight. As such, if you lose weight quickly you will regain back even faster.

There are some health experts who believe that the fast diet and other protocols of intermittent fasting will discourage dieters from healthy eating recommendation such as eating five portions of vegetables and fruits. Another major concern is that the fast diet may trigger binge eating and eating disorders.

Intermittent fasting could cause eating disorders like bulimia and anorexia. This is why healthcare experts often discourage people prone to eating disorders to avoid any fast diets. The fast diet may also not be suitable for underweight individuals.

Others who need to avoid this lifestyle are individuals below the age of 18 years, pregnant and lactating women, anyone recovering from surgery or an illness and those with type 1 diabetes.

Chapter 4: Easy Steps to Get Started

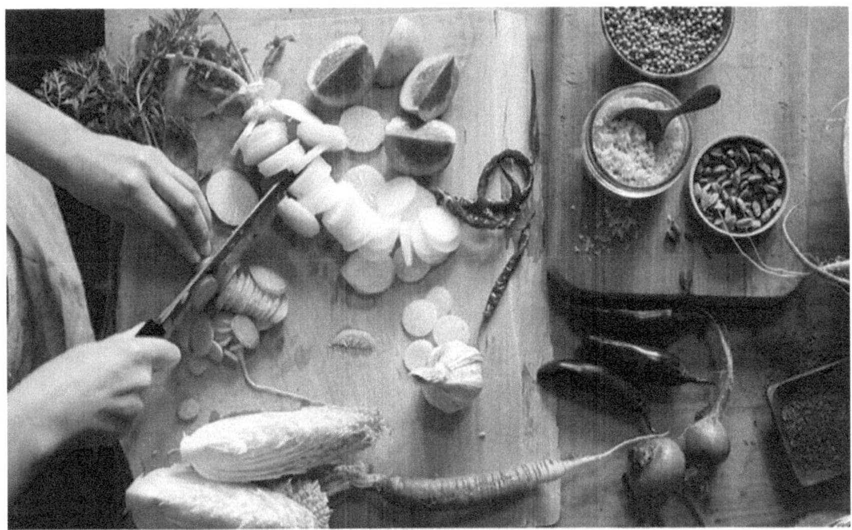

The fast diet is a pretty straightforward diet and lifestyle. It calls for interchanging five days of normal healthy eating with two days of fasting on around 500 and 600 calories. The advantage of this dieting lifestyle is not just shedding of excess weight but also changes the way you look at food and how to lead a healthier, happier life.

In brief, you basically fast for most of the day, usually for 12 to 16 hours and then have the remaining part of your day as an eating window. In this 8 to 12-hour window, you will have all your meals and snacks.

Intermittent fasting is an effective tool for improving your dietary intake. There is plenty of scientific research that supports this diet. It does not have to be unpleasant because there are different approaches to it. In fact, most people who adhere to this lifestyle actually like it and enjoy every single bit of it.

However, on its own, the fast diet won't automatically help you develop lean muscle or achieve optimum fitness goals. You should enhance this diet with regular exercises and healthy eating. This way, it becomes more of a lifestyle than a diet. To be successful, there are a couple of things that you will need to establish.

First, make a determination to follow the fast diet. It simply requires that you fast only 2 days each week. You should then calculate your calories. Basically, you will eat between 500 and 600 calories on your fasting days and between 2200 and 2600 on non-fasting days.

Based on this information, you will then create and follow meal plans that work for you. It is possible to find plenty of healthy, tasty meals that comply with the fast diet that you will enjoy. Then, find workout plans that will work for you.

How to Get Started

Most people divide their calorie intake between breakfast and dinner. It is possible to skip breakfast in order to prolong your fast and then have a more fulfilling and substantial evening meal. The main aim here is to fast for a longer period of time.

- On your fasting days, you will adhere as much as possible to the Fast Diet mantra. This mantra requires that you stick to mostly plant matter and protein. Consume very little carbohydrates. That way, you will stay full for longer and will not need to snack or cheat.

- You should spend some time preparing for your fast days. Think about the kind of meals and snacks you would love to have on these days. This is crucial so that you can then prepare and get them ready. If you do not do this, then you will most likely eat some unhealthy foods like chocolate cake and so on. It is, in fact, advisable to get rid of all of these tempting foods from your refrigerator.

- Learn to stock your house with fast-friendly healthy foods and snacks. They include nuts, dried fruits, sugarless yogurt, salads, and so on. As you fast, and at all other times, drink plenty of water. Water not only hydrates you but it also helps to eliminate toxins in the body. You should also drink water whenever you feel hungry.

- Find a workout pattern that is suitable for you. Plenty of people choose to exercise even on fasting days. Fasted workouts are common because you get to lose even more weight. Teach yourself how to overcome hunger pangs. These will come and disappear. Most of the time we eat because we are stressed or out of boredom. It is rarely because of hunger. If you can learn to eat only during your eating window, then you will fare much better. And remember, even a little bit of real hunger will not kill you.

- Try not to panic or give in whenever you go overboard. For instance, if you eat 600 calories instead of 500 then you should not panic. There is really no magic number out there. It is really just advisable to stick to these numbers as much as possible. However, strict adherence and compliance are not key to success.

- Also, remember to stay positive as you diet. This is a great lifestyle with numerous benefits to your health and wellbeing. Should you fail once or twice, you should not feel discouraged. Sometimes you may not lose any significant weight and may not even feel much better. However, there are long-term goals that you can look forward to and you will lose weight eventually.

Initiate the Following Steps

1. Set out your goals:

You may want to record your current measurements. While this is not compulsory, it is great because you will be able to keep track of your progress with certain goals in mind. Also, check your BMI or body mass index. Your BMI will let you know whether you are within optimum weight for your size or whether you are overweight or even obese. Once you determine your BMI you will then be able to set your weight loss goals. Always ensure that they are realistic. Make sure that your ultimate body weight preference is within the healthy BMI category.

2. Plan to stick to your fast day calorie limit:

The aim of the fast diet is to reduce your daily calorie intake by creating a deficit. If you create a gap between your energy requirements and that which you consume, then your body will burn the difference. We have already seen that the target calorie intake is 500 for women and 600 for men during fasting days. People with higher BMI measurements may find it harder to stick to these limits.

3. Find your two fasting days

When you're choosing your fast days, you need to focus on days when you are not busy and are free from family commitments, pressure, and work-related stress. Keep in mind that your fast day begins after your last evening meal until your next meal the following day. Some of the most popular fast days are Mondays and Wednesdays or Tuesdays and Thursdays. Try and ensure your fast days are not consecutive such as Mondays and Tuesdays. You should only fast on consecutive days once you are used to the lifestyle.

4. Plan your meals and snacks:

It is advisable to plan your meals ahead and prepare ahead of time. The more organized you are then the more likely you are to stay the course and remain faithful to this lifestyle. Plan to eat between 1 and 3 meals on your fast day. You will enjoy greater benefits if the period in between meals is longer. Often, you will find that the later you leave it to eat, the less hungry you will feel. Try and go for green vegetables and lean meats, eggs, and even tofu. You can also have soups, salads, and much more. Basically, the healthier the products the better it is for you.

5. Find a support person or group:

You should ensure that you find a support group or individual that will encourage, support, and share experiences with you. You are definitely more likely to succeed with a support system behind you. There are plenty of credible support groups on different social media sites like Facebook. You will be able to find people who share your interests, passions, and desires.

Additional Steps to Take

- **Count Your Calories**

There are those who say that you do not need to count your calories with intermittent fasting and the fasted diet. This is not accurate because no matter what type of diet you follow calorie count is crucial.

Ideally, if you want to lose weight, then you must take in fewer calories than you burn. On the other hand, if you want to add weight then you should consume more calories than you burn.

The reason why the fast diet is ideal for weight loss and a healthy lifestyle is that you are better able to control your caloric intake. You achieve this better by sticking to the protocol. If you do, then you will see better results in the long run.

How many calories should you be eating?

There are plenty of ways of determining the number of calories that you should eat per meal or per day. Fortunately, there are calorie calculators available online that you can use. You will need to have some personal information handy. For instance, you will need to know your estimated body fat percentage. This is a figure that can be worked out instantly using calculators such as this one. (https://legionathletics.com/how-to-calculate-body-fat)

- Base metabolic rate or BMR
- Activity level
- Lean body muscle
- Total daily energy expenditure

With this information, you will easily be able to calculate the number of calories you should be consuming every day. The most important figure will be the TDEE or total daily energy expenditure.

If you want to lose weight, then you should eat no more than 75 – 80% of TDEE

If you wish to gain weight, then your consumption should be 110 – 115% of TDEE

To simply maintain your weight, then you should eat 100% of TDEE

Macro Nutrient Requirements

Macronutrient dieting is said to be the single most effective tool that you have for managing your body composition. However, this is only when it is applied correctly. While calculations may seem tedious and probably a total waste of time, they are actually worth your time. Therefore, ensure that you are able to work out the correct calorie intake for your needs. And once you get used to it, the process of working out your macronutrients gets even easier.

- **Calculate Macronutrients**

You also need to learn how to calculate your macronutrients. This is crucial especially if you wish to lose fat and not muscle. The same is true if you wish to gain muscle rather than fat. The genesis here is that calories are not identical. Some calories are actually more important than others. Here are some examples that demonstrate this.

- Eating sufficient amounts of carbohydrates helps with workouts and muscle gain.
- Consuming sufficient amounts of proteins helps with recovery, controls, hunger, preserves muscles during workouts, and promotes greater muscle gain.
- Sufficient levels of fats in your diet supports nutrient absorptions, promote a healthy hormone profile, and healthier hair and skin.

Therefore, as you embark on the 5:2 fast diet, you should not just focus on the total calorie count but the calorie type and quality. When we talk about the macros, we are basically referring to the right amounts of fat, carbs, and proteins. You need to be able to work out the right amounts of each that you need to take.

Protein intake

Let us say that your aim is to shed some pounds, and then you need to consume about 1 or 1.2 grams of protein for each pound of body weight a day in order to get the best results.

For instance, if you are overweight or obese, it means that you have about 25% body fat for men and 30% for women. To lose weight, then you will need to reduce your protein consumption to 1 gram per pound of lead muscle mass.

To gain muscle and not lose weight, you should consume 1 gram of protein per pound of overall body weight each day.

Fat intake

If you wish to adjust your diet for fat loss, then you need to eat between 0.2 and 0.25 grams of fat for each pound of body weight every day. However, for maintenance purposes only, then your intake should increase to between 0.3 and 0.35 grams of fat per pound of body weight per day.

Carbohydrate intake

Carbohydrate should constitute the remainder of your calories which is between 30% and 50%. It is easier to work out the exact requirements using a caloric calculator even though you can as well work this out manually.

- **Meal Planning**

Now that you know how to work out your macronutrients, you need to find the right foods and learn how to prepare your meals. Without the right foods at home, you could easily jeopardize your efforts to build a strong healthy body with lean muscle and very little fat. If you can find the best kinds of foods, then you will see results with some basic workouts.

Planning your meals is absolutely crucial. Meal planning refers to making plans for your next meal. It involves planning the food that you will eat and the time that you will eat. It is simply a plan for what you are going to eat and when.

You do not have to make it prohibitive or restrictive at all. As a matter of fact, a suitable meal plan should be all-inclusive rather than restrictive. This way, you will look forward to meal times and will be able to enjoy the nutritious foods that help you achieve your health and weight goals.

Meal Planning Tips

1. Correctly calculate your daily calorie intake

If you want to gain or lose weight, then your efforts will only be effective if you pay attention to your calorie intake. Experts believe that you can lose some weight in the short term if you do not count your calories. However, this strategy is not effective in the long term. For effective weight loss and muscle gain, you really should plan your meals and count your calories.

When you do this, you will free yourself from worry and eat freely without guilt. You will be able to eat the foods that you actually want to eat. It is also empowering knowing the exact results to expect at the end of each week and each month. It all boils down to the energy balance which is the relationship between the calories you consume and those that you burn.

The energy equation

Whenever you set out to achieve something, you should know how to separate the negotiable portions from the non-negotiable ones. This means finding the fundamentals and understanding how to apply them effectively. By doing this you will be able to achieve your goals.

The fundamental principle when it comes to dieting is that if you wish to lose weight, then you must feed your body fewer calories than it burns. A calorie deficit will result in stored fat slowly being whittled down. This fact has been proven to be true by numerous controlled weight loss studies conducted over the last hundred years. These systems include numerous systematic reviews and meta-analyses.

Maintaining calorie deficit for a considerable period of time will result in reduced body fat. However, you should not starve yourself even though weight loss diets urge dieters to eat very little. If you starve yourself, then you will experience negative side effects such as irritability, excessive muscle loss, and metabolic slowdown.

For our purposes, you should endeavor to feed your body about 21 – 25% fewer calories than it expends each day. When you follow this approach, then you will be able to lose from half a pound to as much as 2 pounds each week. You will also be providing your body with all the nutrients that it requires. Again by following this approach, you will preserve your energy levels, metabolic health, mood, hormone production, and overall well-being.

Calorie calculators

There are calculators out there that you can use to work out your caloric requirements. Therefore, before starting out, use one of these modern online calculators in order to find out with high accuracy the amount of energy that you expend each day.

The calculator is likely to give you three different outputs including BMR, LBM, and TDEE. The crucial figure that we seek is TDEE or total daily energy expenditure. In order to determine your energy intake, you will multiply you TDEE by a factor of 0.75 in order to determine your best caloric intake for weight loss.

At this rate, you will have a 25% caloric deficit which indicates the rate at which you will lose fat. This is the recommended approach for weight loss. The situation is different if you wish to gain muscle. Muscle growth requires a different approach which means you will probably have to eat more proteins and basically a lot more food. The reason for this is pretty simple.

Muscle growth is a huge factor of calorie intake and specifically protein consumption. Basically, if you do not consume sufficient amounts of calories then you will most likely not gain muscle. To effectively build muscle, you need to make sure that you are not in a calorie deficit but a surplus instead.

In fact, for purposes of building muscle, you need to consume more calories than the body needs. This is referred to as calorie surplus or positive energy balance. The purpose of the surplus is to ensure your muscles grow unhindered. If you do not work out regularly or stay active then you may add on extra fat as well as muscle mass.

Therefore, if you are building muscle, then you need to know your calorie requirement. We use the same calculator and obtain the same parameters as before. However, in this case, you will multiply your TDEE by 1.1. This will create a 10% caloric surplus and take you to 110% of TDEE.

You need to ensure that you calculate your macronutrients correctly. Remember that the quality of your calories matters. Calorie count on its own won't mean much if it is not good quality. Therefore, avoid junk food and processed foods. Opt for healthy natural options as much as possible.

Even then, remember two things about food. There are no weight loss or weight gain foods. Foods consist of calories in different amounts and have varying macronutrient profiles. Understanding these two factors will aid your weight loss and bodybuilding ambitions.

Generally, foods that are suitable for weight loss are low in calories but rather high in volume and satiating. For instance, whole grains, lean meats, vegetables, fruits, and low-fat dairy.

On the other hand, foods ideal for weight gain is relatively low in volume, high in calories and filling. These foods include pasta, rice, bread, and starches, refined grains, bacon, low-fiber fruits, and so on.

Working Out in a Fasted State

One of the most effective ways of losing weight is to work out in a fasted state. This means working out during your fasting window. However, this is an option and not really a requirement of the 5:2 fast diet.

A lot of people following this lifestyle also prefer doing fasted training. Fasted training basically refers to training during your fasting window. The purpose of this approach is to help you lose weight at a much faster rate.

Fasted training is when you exercise after having fasted for 5 to 6 hours. At this stage, your insulin levels are very low, yet the body is relying on stored energy to keep going.

When you work out after eating, then this is referred to as fed training. During fed training, your insulin levels are high and your body will, therefore, access energy without having to dig into reserves.

Fasted training is not necessary and not even recommended. It is simply an option that you have. You may choose to exercise it or ignore it. It only speeds up your weight loss.

Preference

Most people who follow the fast diet prefer to work out in the morning upon waking up. They choose to work out in the fasted state then prolong their fast till the afternoon when they have their first meal. Some prefer to add some supplements in order to burn even more fats.

There are lots of people across the world looking for ways to gain lean muscle and lose weight in a short period of time. Trainers, health experts, nutritionists, and dieticians now recommend intermittent fasting and specifically the fast diet as the ultimate solution.

Fasted training and the fast diet are excellent ways of structuring your meals and supporting your weight loss goals.

Chapter 5: Simple, Healthy Meal Plans

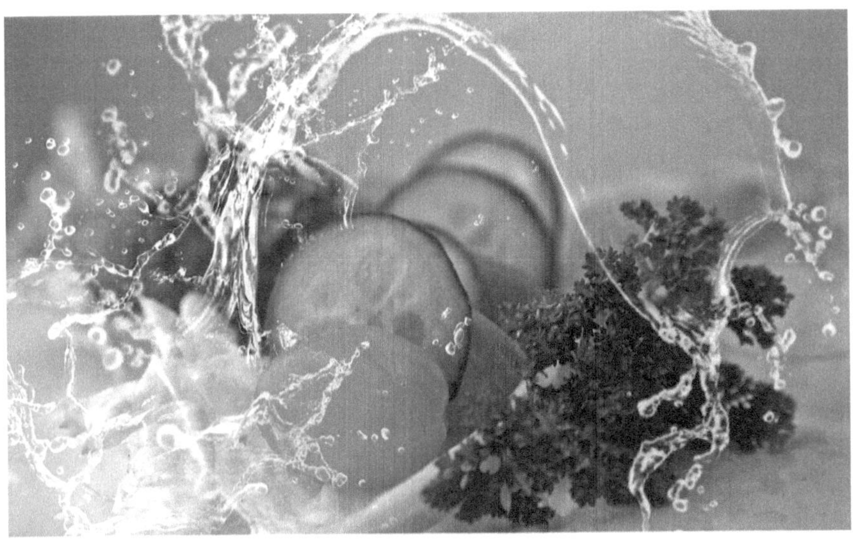

If you choose the 5-2 fast diet lifestyle, then you will choose 2 fasting days when you will fast and limit your calorie intake. For the rest of the days, you will eat normally.

According to dieters who follow this lifestyle, the fast days are the toughest because your calorie intake is limited to only 500 calories for women and 600 calories for men. Surviving on just 500 calories can be tough at first. However, it definitely gets easier with time. You will also feel better if you focus on the benefits that this diet has to offer.

You do not have to eat flat, boring, and tasteless meals simply to keep healthy. There are plenty of options available for healthy yet delicious recipes, meal plans, and tips. It is possible to eat healthily and still enjoy your meals. These delicious meals will ensure that you can comfortably follow this lifestyle without dreading meal times.

Always plan ahead

It does not mean that things will be easy. If you plan your day well complete with meal plans and shopping lists, then you will make it much easier for yourself. On your fast days, you will only consume 500 calories while on your non-fast days you will consume anywhere between 2200 – 2600 calories. Following a diet does not mean that you should miss out on your favorite foods. You can include all your preferred foods, dishes, and snacks.

Meal Planner Samples – 500 Calories or Less

Breakfast – 94 calories
>*Breakfast - 94 calories*

Almonds, Greek yogurt, Sultanas
>Spinach omelet

Lunch - 180 calories
>*lunch – 140 calories*

Mashed potatoes and shoots
>chicken soup

Supper – 170 calories
>*supper – 240 calories*

Chinese vegetable chow
>Moroccan root & couscous

Snacks – 42 calories
>*snack – 27 calories*

½ a cup of almonds
     dried fruit snack

Breakfast for Fast Days

1. Bread and honey – total 95 calories

For breakfast, you will have 1 slice of whole meal bread and two teaspoons of honey. There are 55 calories in the slice of bread and 40 in the honey for a total of 95 calories. This meal is sweet, soft, light, and delicious. It is also quite light.

2. A boiled egg – total 100 calories

A boiled egg is ideal for breakfast. It is packed full of nutrients including vitamins and proteins. The egg will keep you full until your next meal. Sprinkle it with salt and pepper for added taste. This low-calorie breakfast is very simple to make.

3. Chopped kiwi, Greek yogurt, and blueberries – total 95 calories

On day three you will have 1 chopped kiwi, a handful of berries, and half a cup of yogurt. The chopped kiwi has a total of 42 calories with 24 calories for the yogurt and 29 calories for the blueberries. This is a delicious breakfast that is nutritious and satisfying.

4. Mushroom and scrambled egg – total 91 calories

Scrambled eggs are ideal for breakfast because the protein will keep you satisfied all morning. You should, however, avoid any butter or milk. Also, ensure that you have only one egg. You can add some mushroom to add taste and flavor to the egg. A medium size egg has 78 calories while 100 grams of chopped mushrooms have only 12 calories.

5. Watermelon – total of 96 calories

You can also choose to have watermelon fruit for breakfast. Watermelon is nutritious and contains plenty of natural sugars. 300 grams of watermelon contains a total of 96 calories. This offers you a much better option compared to a cereal bar or other breakfast cereals.

6. Almonds, Greek yogurt, and Sultanas – total of 94 calories

A lovely breakfast for your fast day can include Greek yogurt, whole almonds, and a tablespoon of sultanas. There are about 24 calories in 3 tablespoons of fat-free yogurt, 42 calories in one tablespoon of sultanas, and 28 calories in 4 whole almonds. Almonds are full of natural fats while the sultanas provide a whole burst of flavors.

7. Honey and bananas – a total of 99 calories

You will need half a teaspoon of honey with 10 calories and 1 medium sized banana that has a total of 89 calories. Chop up the banana into chunks inside a small bowl and then drizzle it with honey. This simple snack is suitable for breakfast, especially on your fast days. You can warm it in the microwave if you prefer to have it warm.

8. Greek yogurt, apricot, and mixed berries – a total of 96 calories

This breakfast consists of 3 tablespoons of Greek yogurt (24 calories), 1 fresh apricot (17 calories), 50 grams of blackberries (20 calories) 50 grams of strawberries (16 calories), and 50 grams of blackberries (19 calories). Not only will the berries cause your yogurt to last longer but will provide you with the food nutrition that you need and keep you feeling full for a long time.

9. Spinach Omelet – total of 94 calories

Omelets are rich in protein and therefore a great choice for breakfast. A medium egg has 78 calories while 60 grams of spinach contains 16 calories. Beat the egg in a cup and pour onto a pan on medium heat. Once the bottom part is nicely cooked, pour in the spinach and then grill the omelet. Add some salt, some herbs, and pepper to add flavor for a tasty breakfast.

10. Porridge – total of 99 calories

Make porridge using water, a pinch of cinnamon, 30g of porridge oats (89 calories), and ½ a teaspoon of honey (10 calories). Oat porridge is a slow-energy releasing carb and an excellent way to get your day started. The porridge will keep you feeling full for longer. Use water instead of milk to keep the calorie levels low. The cinnamon will add some sweetness to the porridge so remember to add some.

11. Beans on toast – total of 97 calories

This breakfast mill will include 50 grams of baked beans (42 calories) and a slice of wholemeal bread (55 calories). A crusty slice of wholemeal bread with delicious baked beans provides you with a nice start to any day. You should first heat the beans in a microwave then toast the bread. It is a simple yet filling meal.

12. Ham Omelet – total of 97 calories

You will need a thin slice of ham (19 calories) and a medium egg (78 calories). This breakfast meal will take you a total of five minutes to prepare. First, beat the egg in a cup then pour into onto a pan on medium to low heat. As the egg cooks, pour in the chopped ham slice. You can chop the ham into smaller pieces so as to spread the flavor more evenly. This breakfast meal is not just tasty but will keep you from feeling hungry the entire morning.

13. Peanut butter, guava, and banana smoothie – total of calories 130 calories

Take a whole banana and chop it up into a blender. Add some guava and peanut butter. Blend these together for about 3 to 5 minutes. You will then have a delicious and healthy smoothie to take you through the entire morning.

14. Almond butter toast and lemonade – total of 300 calories

Toast a slice of wholemeal bread and spread some almond butter on top. Sprinkle with cinnamon. Prepare a glass of lemonade to down the toast for a healthy and nourishing breakfast.

15. Bowl of dried fruit and nut – 190 calories

Enjoy a bowl of mixed fruit and nut in the morning with a cup of coffee or black tea. Not only will you receive the nourishment you need but will also enjoy the tasty nuts that will keep you feeling full longer.

16. Jaffa cakes – total of 200 calories

Jaffa cakes taste great yet they are low in calories and contain just one gram of fat per cake. Enjoy these tasty cakes with your morning beverage such as black coffee.

Breakfast for Non-Fasting Days

1. Greek Yogurt and Sweet Plums - total of 145 calories per serving

You will need 2 plums (60 calories), 1 teaspoon of honey (20 calories), and 100 grams of low-fat natural yogurt. Simply pour the yogurt into a cup or bowl, add the plums and then top it with honey.

2. Muesli Breakfast Biscuits – total of 228 calories per serving

Muesli contains oats and honey and is very filling. It is a suitable breakfast meal for your mornings and will keep you going till your next meal.

3. Soft boiled egg and asparagus – total of 90 calories per serving

Simply boil a medium size egg (70 calories) then prepare some asparagus (20 calories) for a light yet nutritious breakfast.

4. Low-fat yogurt and banana – total of 177 calories per serving

Enjoy a banana (112 calories) with 100 grams of low-fat natural yogurt (65 calories) for your breakfast. You can add a sprinkle of cinnamon to make it sweeter.

5. Weight Watchers Blueberry Buttermilk Pancakes – total of 206 calories

Blueberries are nutritious while the pancakes are very filling. Enjoy the weight watchers pancakes and lose weight in the process.

6. Carrot, Apple, and Ginger Smoothie – 107 calories per serving

Chop up an apple (55 calories), raw ginger, and 1 carrot (52 calories) and blend them in a blender to produce a delicious smoothie.

7. Bowl of mixed berries – total of 115 calories per serving

Grab a bowl and mix a variety of berries including 100 grams of blueberries (57 calories), 100 grams of raspberries (28 calories)

8. Fruit and nut muesli oat bar – total of 190 calories per serving

Have a muesli oat bar with loads of fruits and nuts. The nuts and oats are low glycemic by nature which means they release energy slowly. You will feel full for a long time after having this breakfast.

9. Almonds and blueberries – total of 157 calories per serving

Enjoy almond nuts and berries for breakfast. You will receive the nutrition that your body requires, keep off the calories, and get the energy that you need for the morning.

10. Banana, peanut butter and chia seeds on toast – 220 calories per serving

Toast a slice of wholemeal bread then spread some peanut butter and sprinkle it chia seeds. Chia seeds are rich in minerals and nutrients. Enjoy with a glass of fresh juice or a cup of coffee.

11. Savory oatmeal with a poached egg – 222 calories per serving

Oatmeal is excellent for getting you off to a great start. You'll receive 150 calories from the oatmeal and 72 calories from the poached egg. The poached egg will provide you with proteins while the oatmeal will keep you full for a long time.

12. Macadamia Ricotta cheese with tomato toast – 190 calories per serving

This is a healthier version of your morning breakfast. Have one slice of tomato toast with homemade ricotta cheese. Ensure that the bread is made out of whole wheat flour. Also, make sure that you use only fresh tomatoes.

13. Egg breakfast muffins – total of 200 calories per serving

Egg breakfast muffins are delicious yet contain very little sugar. They are easy to bake yet very filling. Beat eggs and blend with cheese, some spinach, and bacon. Pour this mixture onto a tray and place it in a preheated oven. The muffins will bake for 25 minutes after which they are ready to serve.

14. Peanut butter and banana smoothie – total of 198 calories per serving

Smoothies are delicious and very filling. You can enjoy this delicious breakfast any day. Simply blend yogurt, honey, soy milk, bananas, and peanut butter. Once the blend is ready, pour it into cups and its ready to serve.

Lunch Meals for Fast Days

1. Quorn Lunch Bowl – total of 165 calories per serving

Quorn is the perfect lunch meal as it is much lower in calories and fat compared to meat and other meals. You can mix quorn with spinach leaves and tender beans. You can produce a lovely stew that takes about 25 minutes to prepare.

2. Chicory, steak, and orange salad – total of 179 calories per serving

Salads do not have to be bland. This specific recipe brings together red onions, a dicey orange, slices of steak, and Dijon mustard. This carb-free meal has no rice, bread, or pasta. This helps bring down the calorie count.

3. Crushed new potatoes, quail eggs, and shoots – total of 170 calories per serve

You can have the occasional carbohydrate even as you fast. Crushed new potatoes go very well with greens and eggs. Opt for quail eggs which are rich in proteins and other nutrients. Add plenty of greens to your meal for a nourishing meal. This meal will keep you full until dinner time.

4. Spring vegetable soup – a total of 163 calories per serving

If you want a healthy lunch, then opt for this nourishing soup. It is a great choice as it is easy to prepare and store. Add loads of vegetables such as carrots, leeks, onions, and so much more. This soup is even better when freshly made at home.

5. Leek and potato soup – total of 134 calories per serving

Soup is a great option for lunch. It does not necessarily have to be a broth. This leek and potato soup is thick and creamy and can be prepared with additional vegetables and seasoning.

6. Chicken pitas – a total of 162 calories per serving

Chicken pitas are low in calories. This meal with skinless chicken, wholemeal pittas, and natural yogurt combine together for a nutritious lunchtime meal. With a side salad of fresh lettuce and tomatoes, you will not just enjoy your meal but receive the nutrition that you need for the afternoon.

7. Crushed potato salad – 200 calories per serving

Prepare a potato salad and include mustard, capers, and gherkins. These will add plenty of flavors to the salad. This is an easy meal to prepare and will save you time. Prepare a large batch and store some for another day.

8. Prawn and fruit cocktail – 130 calories per serving

If you want a lunchtime meal with a difference then have a prawn cocktail with grapes and apples. Now add some fromage frais dressing which is fat-free and full of natural goodness. The dressing replaces the calorie-rich traditional mayo sauce.

9. Creamed corn salad – total of 154 calories per serving

You will need shallots, cream, and sweet corn for this filling and delicious recipe. Cream corn salad is pretty simple and quick to prepare. It also tastes pretty good yet is rather low on calories. You can add some pumpkin seeds and fresh leaves before serving.

10. Pickled cucumber and prawn salad – 100 calories per serving

You will never go wrong with salads particularly at lunchtime. Homemade salads are definitely the best. Prepare your prawns and then add some cucumber. You will enjoy this delicious salad topped with a handful of ingredients.

11. Artichokes and Spanish tortilla – total of 107 calories per serving

Protein is an ideal nutrient for health and eggs provide one of the best sources. Eggs also keep you full for longer so that you do not have to snack between meals. Use tender artichokes and medium size eggs with some parsley to add flavor.

12. Chicken miso soup – 132 calories per serving

This is yet another very simple soup to prepare. It takes only 10 minutes to prepare yet is very healthy. This soup is also ideal if you are trying to lose weight because it consists mostly of water. Add some mushrooms and ginger for increased flavor.

13. Tarka Dhal – 137 calories per serving

Tarka is a delicious Indian lentil that is great for your lunch meal. While it is normally served as a side dish, it is so tasty and nutritious that you can have it on its own. You need only a handful of ingredients to enjoy a wonderful lunch meal.

14. Assorted bean salad with mustard dressing – 180 calories per serving

Beans provide you with lots of protein and fiber. They also fill you up so you stay full until time for your next meal. This meal includes a variety of beans including borlotti, cannellini, and green. Adding some mustard adds a tasty flavor to this dish.

15. Warm cabbage salad – 129 calories per serving

If you want to have a light lunch, then consider having this cabbage salad. It will fill you up sufficiently and you will enjoy the varied taste of the added pumpkin seeds, fennel, and mustard. You will love the flavors and will also benefit from the proteins, vitamins, and all other nutrients.

Lunch Meals for Non-Fast Days

1. Chicken drumsticks roast – 342 calories per portion

Chicken is low in calories but very filling and loaded with proteins. Take a serving of chicken drumsticks and roast in the oven. Chicken drumsticks are much healthier than thighs and breasts because of the little fat they have on the bone. You will remain full after this meal for a long while.

2. Seafood soup – 295 calories per serving

This delicious soup is very filling and suitable for lunch on regular, non-fast days. This stock is made using tender prawns and a variety of spices. The stock is prepared right from scratch and is a lot healthier compared to cream-based ingredients. You can use fresh lemongrass sticks to add more flavor.

3. Spinach and stuffed chicken – 277 calories per portion

One of the most delicious yet filling meals is stuffed chicken and spinach. This meal is low in calories and is prepared by roasting it in the oven without adding any oil. Stuff the chicken with fresh spinach and then serve with a variety of vegetables. This is an excellent meal that will keep you from snacking the rest of the day.

4. Roast haddock – 350 calories per portion

Fish is an excellent choice if you want a tasty yet filling and nutritious meal. All you will need is fresh haddock, veggies, and some balsamic vinegar. This meal is very low in calories and fats yet high in nutrition and very tasty.

5. Tuna pasta – 349 calories per portion

This is a healthy and rather light meal suitable for your lunch. Use medium-sized fresh tuna chunks to prepare this meal and not the tinned version. Tuna is packed full of protein and. Enjoy this low fat creamy sauce for a guilt-free and filling meal any afternoon.

6. Tomato, artichoke, and red onion pizza – 310 calories per portion

A homemade pizza is much healthier and probably tastier than a commercially produced one. Avoid pizza dough and use tortillas instead for the base. You will reduce the calorie count immensely. Fresh vegetables and homemade tomato sauces add rich natural flavors to this meal.

7. Duck and noodle stir-fry – total of 290 calories per portion

If you want a quick, easy, and cheap meal, then this is exactly what you want. Duck breast is low in fat and tasty when properly prepared. Prepare the noodles separately and add a dash of soy sauce. Then stir fry with duck breasts and enjoy a fantastic meal that is great any time of any day.

8. Bean, mince, and mash pie – 350 calories per serving

This pie is less than 400 calories yet it combines plenty of veggies with lean beef mince together with a homemade tomato sauce. You will enjoy this guilt-free meal which is not just filling but also very healthy. It is even healthier when you swap pie toppings with mash instead of pastry.

9. Butternut squash Risotto – total of 310 calories per serving

This low-fat risotto is low on calories and has very few ingredients. You will only need to use stock, rice, and low-fat butternut squash. This is a low-fat meal suitable for your lunchtime meal. It is also very filling and will leave you satiated until your next meal. To keep the fat levels even lower, use spray oil.

10. Low-calorie chicken tikka masala – 392 calories per serving

If you love chicken masala, then you will truly enjoy this chicken tikka masala. This homemade version is much better than anything you can buy at a fast food outlet. It has 36% less fat compared to others so you will consume fewer calories and still enjoy your delicious meal.

11. Leek, pea, and mint-stuffed lamb – 300 calories per portion

This is an amazing lunch option especially for weekends when the family is around. The stuffed lamb is full of juicy flavors. It is stuffed with fresh peas and mint flavor than roasted in the oven in its own juices for some of the most amazing flavors. There is no added fat but you can sprinkle it with natural spices, salt, and black pepper.

12. Couscous and Moroccan root tagine – maximum of 238 per portion

This is a great meal if it's just you and someone special because it will definitely please and tease your taste buds. It is not just low in calories but also healthy and light. It is made with plenty of veggies and fresh tomato sauce. Serve some root tagine as the main starch as well as couscous which is great for you. It is made of whole wheat and therefore digests slowly in the stomach. The tagine has spicy flavors that you will absolutely love.

13. Squash, stir-fry, and sea bass – for a total of 332 calories per serving

If you love fish for dinner, then you will enjoy this sea bass dinner. It is a simple dish to prepare that is also low in fat. Cut the fish into chunks and cook in a frying pan. Top it with garlic and give it sufficient flavors so that you enjoy this delicious fish without any guilty feelings.

14. Pepper fajitas and pork – total of 276 calories per serving

This is a fajita recipe prepared using crisp peppers and juicy pork meat. This is a really delicious meal that most people can't believe it is less than 400 calories. Season the fajita with plenty of spices, herbs, and other natural seasonings. This way, you will not have to use oil. You should use low-fat yogurt in place of sour cream in order to minimize the calories.

15. Italian fish stew – total calories is 360 per portion

Use fresh fish to prepare this low fat and low-calorie dish. Fresh fish fried in a pan with lots of fish stew and added vegetables including tomatoes, onions, turnips, and so on. Prepare tomato sauce and enjoy this delicious yet nourishing low-fat fish stew.

Even as you limit your calorie intake, the body still needs nourishment. Dinner is one of the most important meals of the day. Therefore you should focus on what you eat as well as calorie intake. Here are some meals that you can have on both your fast and non-fast days. It is important to count calories because the main reason why we add or lose weight is through calories we eat.

Dinners for Fast Days

1. Green miso noodle bowl – total of 198 calories per serving

This delicious noodle soup contains lots of herbs and fresh vegetables. It is easy to prepare and is low in calories. This meal takes 2 minutes to prepare and 8 minutes cooking time. The mixture of fresh vegetables and herbs will provide you with numerous nutrients that you need. The meal is low in calories, hence why you can eat until full without any worries or guilt.

2. Roasted ratatouille – has 150 calories per serving

This meal consists of large chunks of vegetables in a freshly prepared tomato sauce. It is a meal that contains a large variety of nutrients from minerals to vitamins as well as phytonutrients and macronutrients. It contains delicious vegetables such as bell peppers, aubergines, and courgettes.

3. Fast fish burger – 143 calories per portion

The main dish in this meal is the low-calorie, nutritious, white fish fillets. Preparing the fish fillet is easy and takes only five minutes. Use a wholemeal or whole-wheat bun to prepare the burger and stuff with lots of onions, tomatoes, and bell peppers. Eat this burger with a side dish of vegetables. The bun is not included in the calorie count.

4. Mediterranean vegetable chili – total of 195 calories per portion

This vegetable chili contains a sufficient quantity of vegetables. They include cherry tomatoes, courgettes, aubergines, and spinach. You can also add kidney beans and spices to make the meal more tasty and nourishing.

5. Chinese vegetable chow – 170 calories per serving

This is a Chinese meal that is actually less than 200 calories. It contains delicious healthy ingredients including oyster sauce, rice vinegar, a light soy and plenty of vegetables. It also contains egg noodles which contain lots of essential proteins. This is a very tasty meal that will leave you feeling nice and full for a long time.

6. Prawn curry – 194 calories

This is the Vietnamese prawn curry that takes only 15 minutes to prepare. Take the prawns and prepare them for the pot. Use a wide variety of vegetables then include a healthy curry with lots of chili peppers. No need to prepare an additional meal as this is very nourishing and filling.

7. Chinese dumplings – 64 calories per servings

A single portion of Chinese dumplings has only 64 calories. Dumplings are very light yet tasty and satisfying. Since the calories are so low, you can have more than one serving or a side dish of noodles. Such a dish consists of an additional 90 calories. Chinese dumplings are easy to prepare and great for a family dinner.

8. Vegetable balti – 131 calories per serving

This vegetable balti contains plenty of vegetables with lots of natural seasoning such as garlic, black pepper, and red bell peppers. Your balti should contain a variety of vegetables such as parsley, tomatoes, courgettes, broccoli, parsnips, butternut squash, and spinach. You can have the vegetable balti with one serving of brown rice which is only 83 calories.

9. Vegetable tagine and spiced butternut squash – total of 150 calories

One of the best ways of having your vegetables is to cook them in a tagine. They will acquire lots of flavors making them tasty and appealing. This is a Moroccan- style casserole with chickpeas that will keep you feeling full all evening. There is no need for a side dish with this meal.

10. Baked aubergine – 81 calories per portion

An aubergine is a purple egg-shaped fruit that makes a very tasty and nutritious meal. They have a nice meaty texture that you will love. Aubergines are also filling which makes them an ideal dinner meal so you won't feel hungry before bedtime. This meal simply takes out the inside of an aubergine, adds plenty of flavors to it, and puts it back.

11. One-pot Italian style mussels – has a total of 220 calories per serving

This meal not only consists of delicious and nutrient-rich mussels but also has olives, anchovies, and garlic. These add flavor to the mussels and enrich the meal. Other ingredients include tomatoes, bay leaves, and white wine. You can enjoy this dish with a slice of wholemeal bread or brown rice.

12. Squash curry and prawns – 291 calories per portion

This is a curry that is so full of flavors you will ask for a second serving. Not only are the prawns delicious and full of healthy oils and protein but there is a good portion of vegetables. The squash, spinach, and basil make this not just a tasty meal but also very nutritious.

13. Asian sea bass – 279 calories per portion

If you love fish then you are lucky because it is among the best sources of animal protein. Fish will also keep you fuller for longer. Fish such as the Asian sea bass contain essential omega 3 fatty acids which are hugely important to the body. Add some chilies, ginger, and sesame oil to infuse goodness, great taste, and an overall healthy meal for your dinner.

14. Moroccan rice-stuffed tomatoes – 211 calories per portion

If you want a simple yet complete meal, then these Moroccan rice-stuffed tomatoes are just right for you. It takes only 25 minutes to prepare. The stuffing includes pine nuts, courgettes, rice, and spices. These beef-steal tomatoes are absolutely tasty and you will definitely love them.

15. Couscous and Moroccan root tagine – 240 calories per portion

This delicious meal is ideal for you because of its numerous ingredients. The couscous contains chickpeas, carrots, and courgettes as well as some veggies. Not only is this meal good for you but is also very tasty. You have naturally spiced tomato sauce that brings the vegetables very well together.

Dinner Meals for Non-Fasting

16. Baked eggs with spinach and mushroom – 270 calories per serving

This dinner meal can also serve as your breakfast. You have soft mushroom, nutrient-rich vitamins, and rich, creamy eggs. On top of this, you also have a light cream sauce that tops up your meal so that you receive the nutrients that your body needs but with very few calories.

17. Root and barley soup – total of 261 calories per serving

Soups may not be ideal for dinner especially if they are light. However, if you add quality ingredients, ensure that the soup is thick, and there is a side dish such as a slice of wholemeal bread. Other ingredients that make this soup so worthwhile include barley, vegetables, and barley. This is the main meal that you will definitely like.

18. Coconut curry and Thai chicken – 283 calories per portion

This delicious Thai dish is an excellent choice for your dinner. The chicken is prepared with fresh, natural spices such as garlic, parsley, rosemary, and tomatoes. The coconut adds an extra taste to make this a sumptuous dinner for you and your household. Have it with a side dish of brown rice.

19. Noodles and Japanese broth – 250 calories per serving

Noodles provide you with the necessary carbs while soup has numerous nutrients. Both are very filling. The beef in the soup is full of flavor from all the seasoning. If you want a sumptuous, low-calorie meal, then this definitely is the one for you.

20. Pork chops with pomegranate and mango salsa – 222 calories per serving

A fruit salsa is definitely a nutritious addition to your meal. Pork meatballs are not just tasty but also full of proteins and trace minerals. Your plate will consist of delicious pork meatballs, pita bread, chunks of mango and pomegranates.

21. Stuffed Chicken with spinach – a total of 277 calories per portion

If you want to eat a healthy yet nutritious meal that will keep you full for longer, then your best option is this stuffed chicken dish with healthy, leafy spinach. It is low in calories yet the stuffed chicken is delicious and enjoyable. The spinach is steamed and seasoned to keep you not just healthy but also happy.

22. Tuna Past – 349 calories per portion

Tuna pasta is a light, healthy, and simple meal. Tuna is packed full of proteins and essential oils such as omega 3 fatty acids. Have this meal with a low-fat creamy sauce so that you enjoy a nutritious, tasty, yet filling meal.

23. Tomato pizza and red onion artichoke – 315 calories per serving

Homemade pizza is healthier than all others. You will use tortillas for the base and not pizza dough which is not healthy at all. Ensure that you have fresh veggies and some great homemade tomato sauce.

24. Roast haddock and steamed veggies – total of 371 calories per serving

This is yet another delicious fish dish. Fish is always a great choice and you can never go wrong. Roast the fish in the oven and sprinkle it with balsamic vinegar, salt, black pepper, garlic and lots of other natural seasonings. A dash of lemon will spruce up the taste. Steam your veggies including some spinach, broccoli, and cabbage leaves.

26. Duck noodle stir-fry – a total of 293 calories per serving

If you are searching for a healthy but affordable option, then go for stir-fry. This particular meal is low in fat but with sufficient natural flavors. Use a shallow pan to fry this meal. It takes about 7 minutes to be ready.

27. Mash, bean, and mince pie – a total of 355 calories

It is possible to find pies that are actually less than 400 calories. This recipe combines lean beef with lots of vegetables and homemade, natural tomato sauce. There are plenty of natural ingredients for the seasoning.

28. Low-fat butternut squash risotto – maximum 320 calories per serving

You will find that this classic low-fat squash risotto has few but powerful ingredients. These include stock, rice, and butternut squash. It is not just low in calories but keeps you satisfied all evening till your next meal.

29. Chicken and barley salad – total of 384 calories

Salads can be interesting especially if you include color and variety. The nice and warm chicken salad has a lot of variety including almonds which are filling and contain essential vitamins. Have this salad with barley rather than rice.

30. Chicken tikka masala – total of 392 calories per serving

If you love curry then you will enjoy this chicken tikka dish. It is a favorite of many including fast dieters. The best part is that this chicken has very little fat compared to other chicken tikkas. The reason is that we do not use oil to prepare the sauce but a fat-free yogurt.

Conclusion

Thanks for making it through to the end of this book. Let's hope it was informative and able to provide you with all of the tools you need to achieve your goals, whatever they may be.

The next step is to get prepared to change your lifestyle by adapting the fast diet. This diet has changed the lives of numerous people. It will help you to lose weight, keep it off, develop lean muscle, look great, feel even better, and generally enjoy your best life.

You will also enjoy great health. Intermittent fasting and especially the fast diet will help to keep chronic diseases and illnesses at bay. Not only will you look good and feel great but you will also enjoy exceptional health.

Finally, if you found this book useful in any way, a review on Amazon is always appreciated!

Other Books By Clarissa Fleming

- Keto Meal Prep For Lazy People: 21-Day Ketogenic Meal Plan to Lose 15 Pounds:
https://www.amazon.com/dp/B07H43V8CH

- Lectin Free Cookbook: No Hassle Lectin Free Recipes In 30 Minutes or Less:
https://www.amazon.com/dp/B07H7T2SVM

- Lectin Free Cookbook: 74 Best Easy Lectin-Free Electric Pressure Cooker Recipes:
https://www.amazon.com/dp/B07F2KGX94

- Freestyle 2018: 105 Best Easy And Healthy Recipes To Quickly Lose Weight:
https://www.amazon.com/dp/B07HRT1R35

- Lectin Free Cookbook: 2 Manuscripts - 74 Best Easy Lectin-Free Electric Pressure Cooker Recipes + No Hassle Lectin Free Recipes In 30 Minutes or Less:
https://www.amazon.com/dp/B07JDNR772

- Keto Fat Bombs For Lazy People: 38 Must-Try Savory and Sweet Ketogenic Fat Bomb Recipes:
https://www.amazon.com/dp/B07K5C4QLJ